Matchstick Mini is Kind to his Family and Friends

By Edel Malone

Original concept created, illustrated, and written by Edel Malone. I'm sure you will love these books as much as I do. I know you will enjoy making lasting memories with your child moving forward in all stages of their lives by encouraging your child to tell you what's on their mind throughout their lifetime. Asking questions is the way forward. Check out the other Matchstick Mini books from this series.

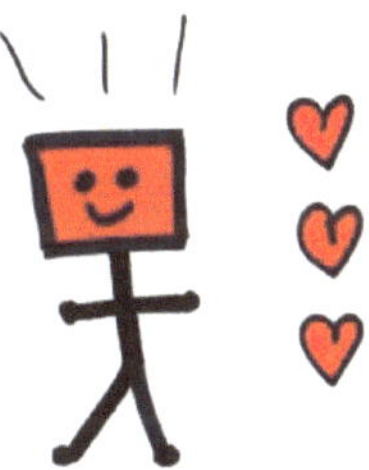

I dedicate these books to all my nieces and nephews. "Matchstick Mini is Kind to his Family and Friends", all rights reserved to Edel Malone, no parts from this book can be used without permission ©copyright 2022 Thank you for buying my book. First edition 2022. For more information contact lifestylethoughtscoaching@gmail.com

The Matchstick Mini book series has been designed to encourage your child to open up and talk about what is on their mind from an early age. The topics covered are related to young children to encourage good communication techniques carrying on into each stage of their lives, keeping safety and values in mind. Sizes and colors may vary for printed books.

OTHER BOOKS FROM MATCHSTICK MINI

Matchstick Mini and Safety

Matchstick Mini and Others

Matchstick Mini has Fun

Matchstick Mini and School

Matchstick Mini is Very Good

Matchstick Mini is Healthy

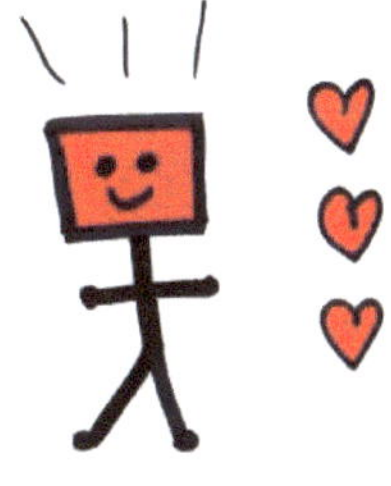

Matchstick Mini always tries to be nice to his family, and they always try to be nice to him too. Matchstick Mini always says please and thank you to them and asks them how their day was. Matchstick Mini always asks his family if they are okay when they are sad or upset, and he always tells someone in his family if he is not okay too.

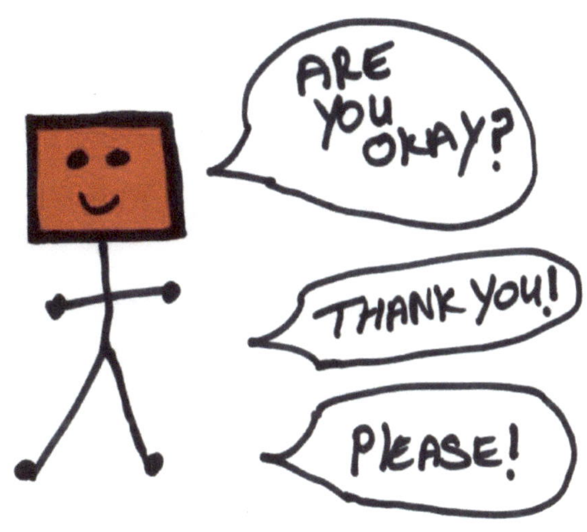
ARE YOU OKAY?
THANK YOU!
PLEASE!

Matchstick Mini likes to help his family around the house and in the garden. He likes to help tidy the garden after a nice sunny day, and he brings his toys, cups, and plates into the house. Matchstick Mini likes to help carry shopping bags into the house when his family go shopping, and he always puts his rubbish in the bin to help around the house, so one person does not have to do everything.

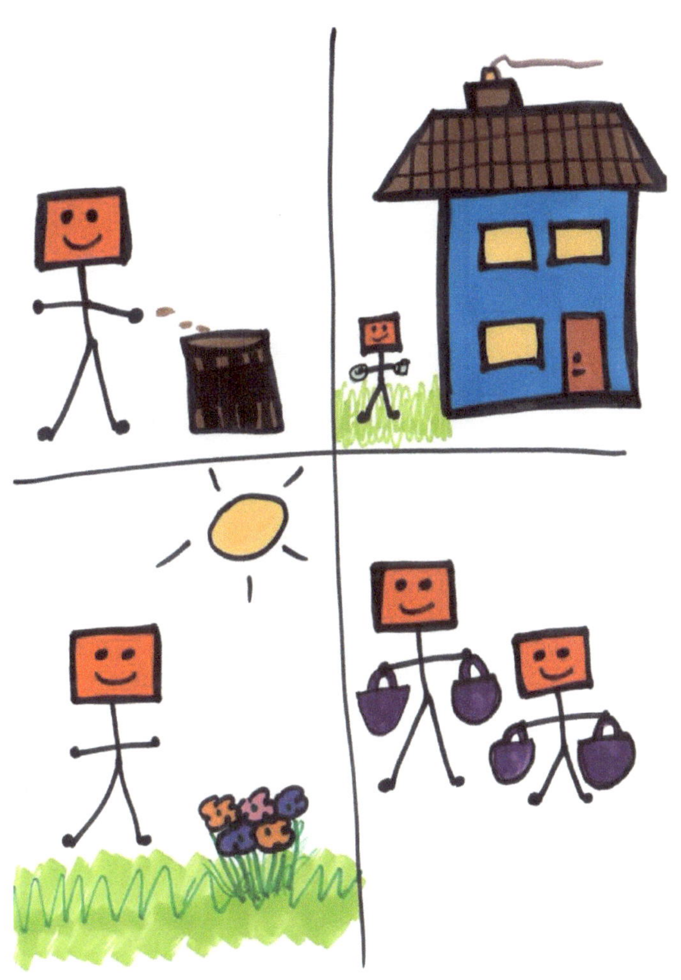

At Christmas and other people's birthdays, Matchstick Mini likes to make birthday cards and Christmas cards for all his family and friends. At Christmas, Matchstick Mini likes to draw Christmas trees on Christmas cards. He draws balloons and hearts on the birthday cards he makes and writes a lovely message. Matchstick Mini likes to be creative and has lots of fun making the cards. Matchstick Mini knows that people like to receive nice cards.

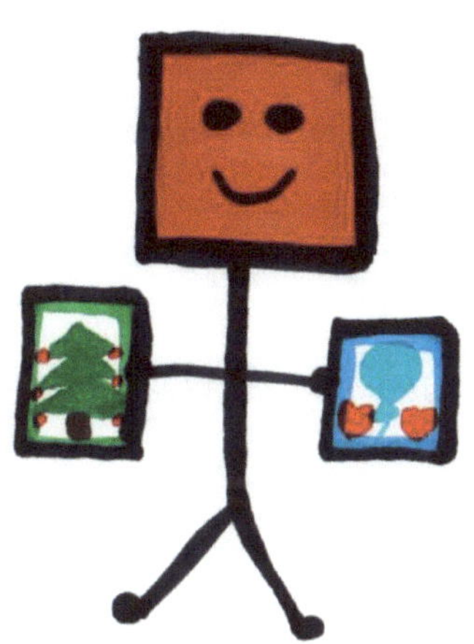

Sometimes Matchstick Mini likes to make presents for other people or buy them presents in the shop. Matchstick Mini loves going to the shop to buy presents, and he loves looking at all the different things in the shop. Matchstick Mini enjoys making presents at home too and he loves to be creative. Do you like to be creative like Matchstick Mini?

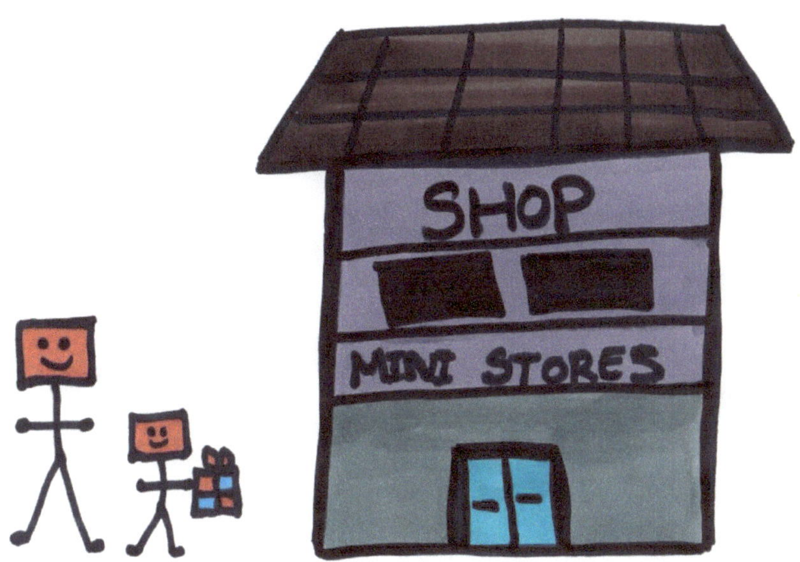

SHOP
MINI STORES

Matchstick Mini always says sorry when he has done something wrong to upset someone in the family. Matchstick Mini knows that sometimes everyone can make mistakes, and he will always say sorry when he makes a mistake. Matchstick Mini is very good, and he cares about how his family feels.

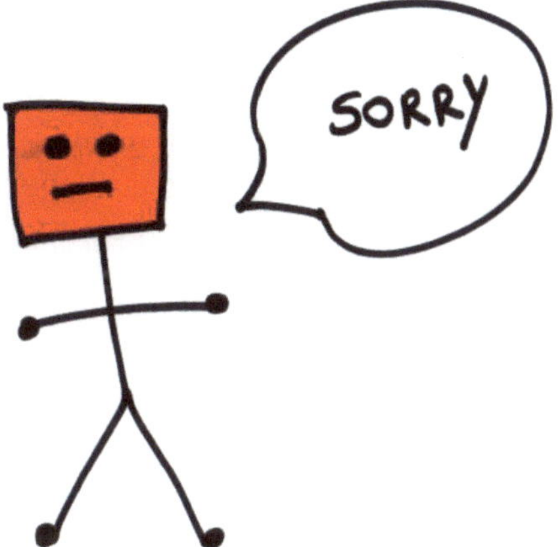
SORRY

Matchstick Mini and his little sister always share, and they like to share with their friends too. Matchstick Mini likes to be nice to his family and friends. Are you always nice to your family and friends, and are they always nice to you?

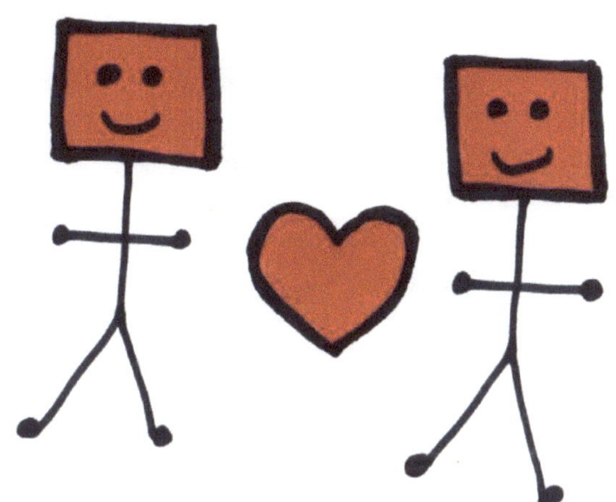

Matchstick Mini always includes his family and friends in his games, he does not like to leave anyone out. Matchstick Mini does not want to be left out of games either. He knows it is not nice to be left out. Does anyone ever leave you out from games?

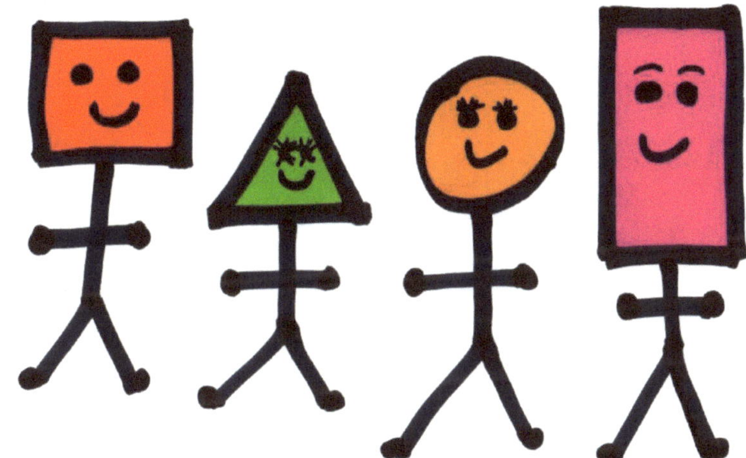

Matchstick Mini won't use bad language towards his family and friends. He knows it is not nice to say bad words to anyone, and he knows he would get into trouble with his teacher in school if he used bad words in school too.

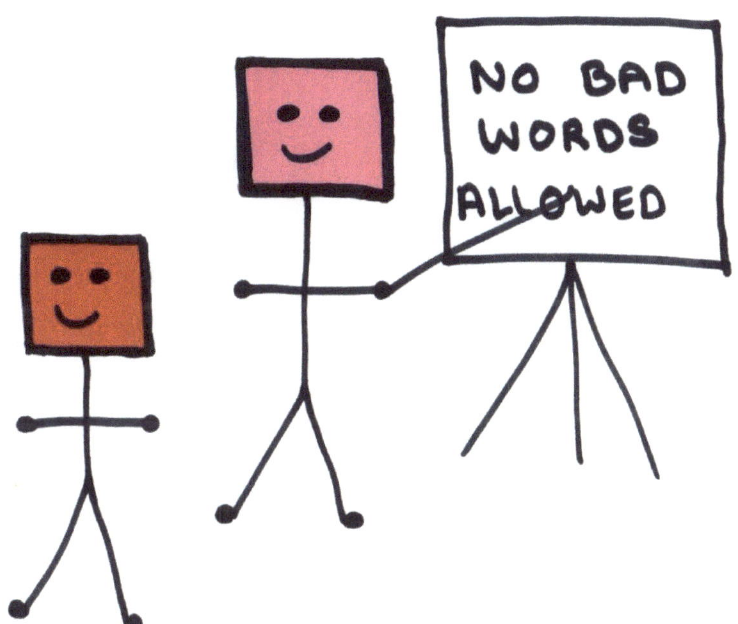

NO BAD
WORDS
ALLOWED

Matchstick Mini won't call his family hurtful names. He knows it is not nice to call other people hurtful names. Matchstick Mini will always tell an adult if someone is calling him names that are not nice, and he will always tell his family if someone has hurt his feelings too. Do you tell an adult if someone is not nice to you?

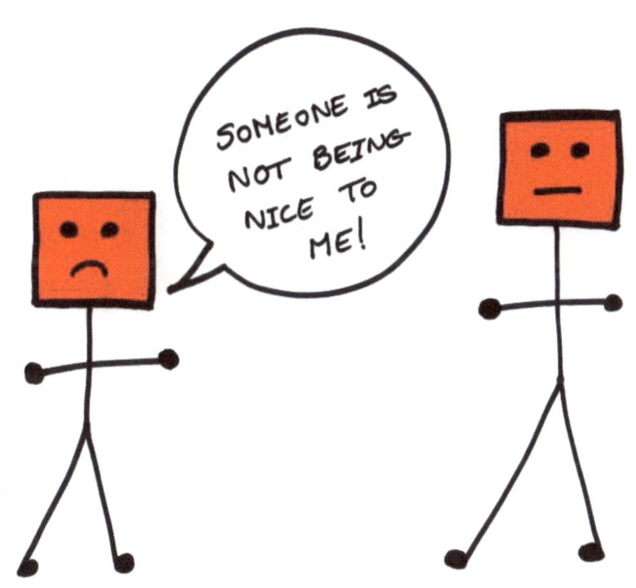
SOMEONE IS NOT BEING NICE TO ME!

Matchstick Mini won't tease his friends or family or be mean to his family in front of his friends. He knows it is not nice, and it can be very hurtful. So Matchstick Mini always tries his best to be nice to everyone. When Matchstick Mini's friends come over to his house, he is nice to his little sister, who loves dressing up as a princess.

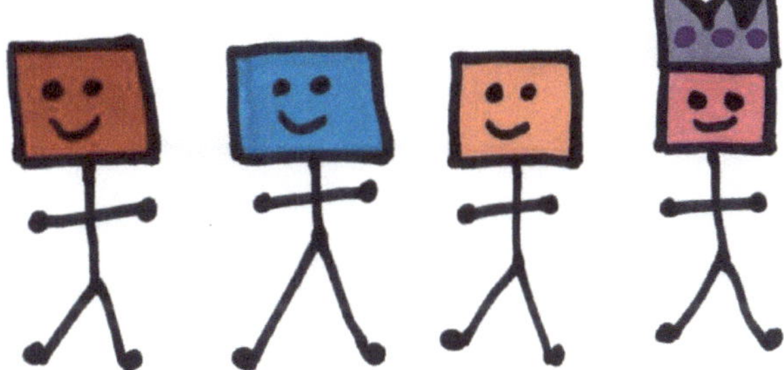

Matchstick Mini loves that his family are all unique and different. He loves that they all sound different and he loves that they all have different personalities and like different things. Do you love that everyone in your family is different from each other, like Matchstick Mini?

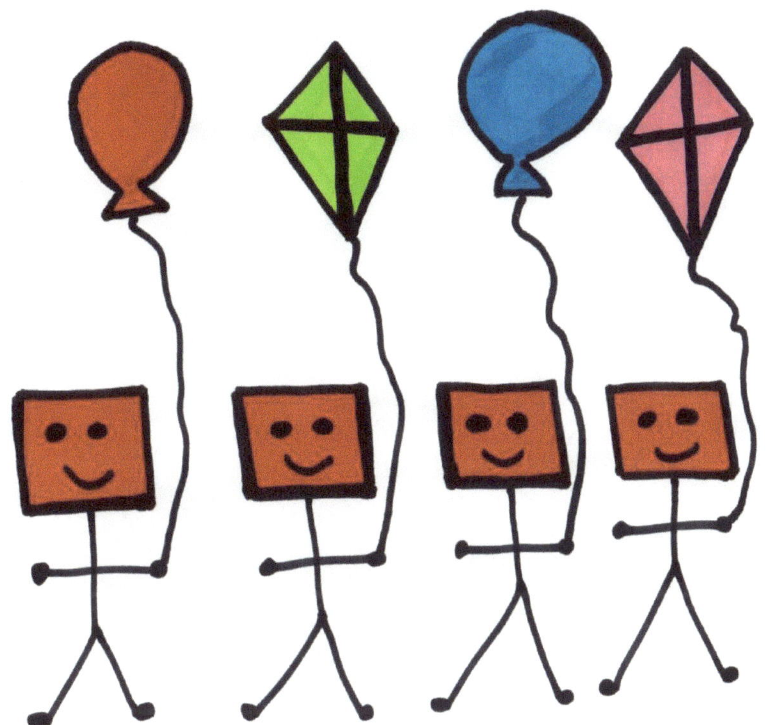

Matchstick Mini has respect for his family and listens to them, and he likes to hear what they have to say. Matchstick Mini waits until someone is finished talking before, he says what he has to say. Do you wait until someone is finished talking before it is your turn to speak like Matchstick Mini?

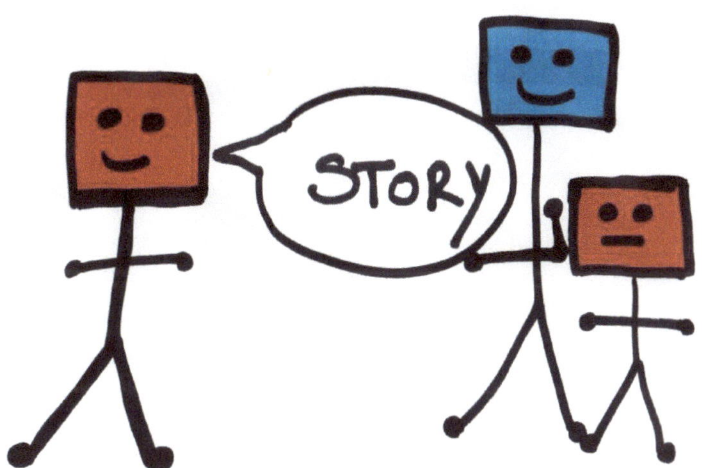
STORY

Matchstick Mini obeys family rules, and he likes to know what acceptable and unacceptable behavior is. Matchstick Mini likes rules, and he knows that rules are there for a good reason and safety. So, what are your family rules? Maybe your family could have a tea party, talk about the rules, and write them down someday.

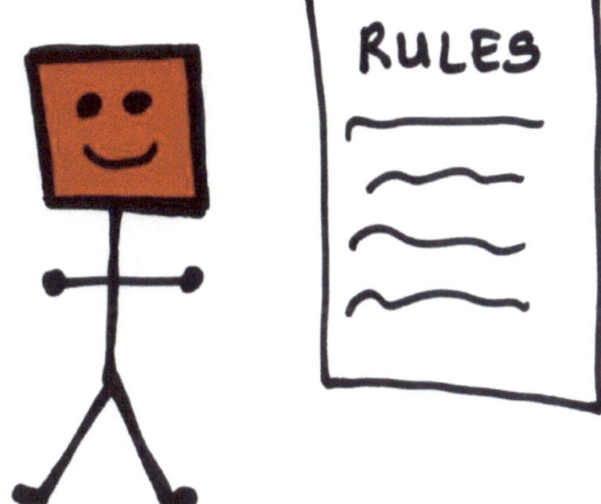

RULES

If one of Matchstick Mini's family members is sick, he looks after them by bringing them drinks. Matchstick Mini asks them if they are okay, and he helps to tidy up. Matchstick Mini tries to be quiet if they are asleep. Matchstick Mini knows sleep, drinking water, hot drinks, healthy food, and plenty of rest helps people get better quickly.

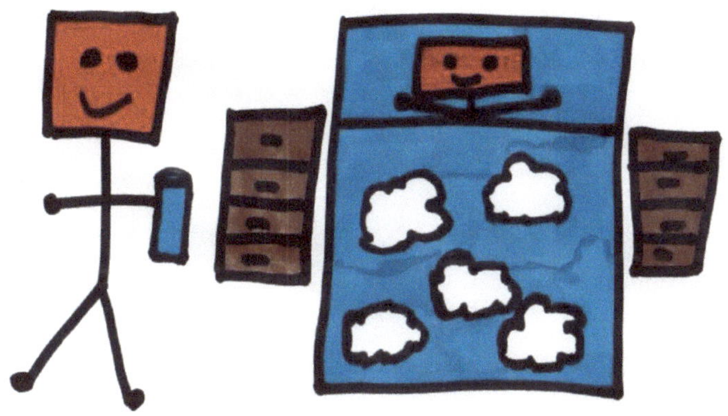

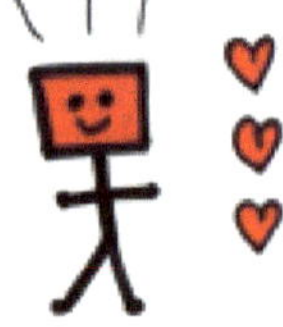